RESETTING YOUR ADRENAL SYSTEM

HOW TO FIGHT ADRENAL FATIGUE SYNDROME, INCREASE YOUR ENERGY AND LOWER STRESS LEVELS

I0449827

BY SMART READS

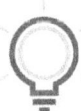

Free Audiobook

As a thank you for being a Smart Reader you can choose 2 FREE audiobooks from audible.com. Simply sign up for free by visiting www.audibletrial.com/Travis to get your books.

Visit:
www.smartreads.co/freebooks
to receive Smart Reads books for FREE

Check us out on Instagram:
www.instagram.com/smart_readers
@smart_readers

ABOUT SMARTREADS

Choose Smart Reads and get smart every time. Smart Reads sorts through all the best content and condenses the most helpful information into easily digestible chunks.

We design our books to be short, easy to read and highly informative. Leaving you with maximum understanding in the least amount of time.

Smart Reads aims to accelerate the spread of quality information so we've taken the copyright off everything we publish and donate our material directly to the public domain. You can read our uncopyright below.

We believe in paying it forward and donate 5% of our net sales to Pencils of Promise to build schools, train teachers and support child education.

To limit our footprint and restore forests around the globe we are planting a tree for every 10 hardcover books we sell.

Thanks for choosing Smart Reads and helping us help the planet.

Sincerely,

Travis & the Smart Reads Team

TABLE OF CONTENTS

INTRODUCTION

In this book, you will learn all you need to know about adrenal fatigue syndrome and the various strategies and treatments available for overcoming this condition.

You may be living a life filled with overwhelming stress. Maybe you struggle with lethargy and focusing on what is happening around you at any given moment. Getting some decent sleep at night could also be a problem for you.

Do any of these descriptions apply to you? If so, then you may be a victim of adrenal fatigue. This syndrome prevents you from handling stress well.

This book will uncover the deep details of adrenal fatigue so that you can finally recover and live a healthy, happy life.

CHAPTER 1: UNDERSTANDING ADRENAL FATIGUE

Each and every one of us has undergone overwhelming stress during our lives. You may believe you are able to manage stress, but your hormones could be telling a different story. Your adrenal glands could be trapped in a cycle that results in severe adrenal fatigue disorder. This may sound scary, but the reality is that there are millions of people all over the world who suffer from this syndrome. It may be a diagnosis that is somewhat contentious, but there are measures you can take to control the symptoms and have a total recovery.

One of the hormones produced by the adrenal glands is cortisol. It helps in controlling stress, and if your adrenal glands fail to release enough of this hormone, then your body won't be able to cope with the daily stresses of life. There are a number of symptoms that can result from this, but the major one is fatigue.

These symptoms can be divided into two categories: the common symptoms that are prevalent in most people, and the uncommon symptoms that only a few suffer from. However, it is possible to exhibit a blend of both.

Common Symptoms:

1. **Difficulty waking up in the morning** – This is a common symptom among people who are undergoing the initial stages of the disease. Due to the overwhelming stress, a person has problems waking up even though they slept well in the night. The stress tends to elevate the adrenaline and cortisol levels, thus disrupting your body's sleep cycle.

2. **Daily fatigue** – During the latter stages of the syndrome, there is a decrease in production of norepinephrine neurotransmitter, cortisol, and adrenaline. This is the reason why people who suffer from the syndrome tend to lack energy all day, though an exception to this does exist, but this will be tackled later on.

3. **Stress** - People who are undergoing the latter stages usually cannot cope with stress due to the depressed levels of neurotransmitters and cortisol. Every time you experience stress, your adrenal glands secrete adequate amounts of norepinephrine, adrenaline, and cortisol to boost awareness and strength to focus on the situation at hand. Without these hormones in adequate quantities, the body fails to respond as it should, causing apathy, irritability, and anxiety.

4. **Craving for salty food** – The adrenal gland has a part called the Cortex, which is designed to produce a hormone known as aldosterone. Aldosterone is responsible for regulating fluid and mineral excretions in conjunction with the kidneys. In cases where the adrenals experience fatigue, inadequate aldosterone is produced, resulting in the majority of vital minerals being flushed out via urination. This is why most people suffering from adrenal fatigue cannot balance their sodium, magnesium, and potassium levels. They end up craving foods that are salty just to replenish what they have lost.

5. **Late energy surge** – Most people experience elevated cortisol levels in the morning, and this decreases as the day progresses. However, a person in the early stages of adrenal fatigue syndrome, whose adrenal glands can still produce high cortisol levels, will tend to be energetic much later on. If you sense you are strangely energetic in the evenings when you have been sluggish throughout the day, then this could be the reason.

6. **Weak immune system** – Another function of cortisol is the reduction of inflammation and thus the regulation of the immune system. Inflammation generally signifies that the body is fending off an infection and is healing itself, and cortisol is supposed

to control this process. If your cortisol levels become elevated due to too much stress, it brings inflammation too low and suppresses your immune system, thus causing weakness in the body. Alternatively, if cortisol levels drop significantly, then the body experiences chronic inflammation or autoimmune diseases.

Uncommon Symptoms:
1. Dizziness
2. Painful joints
3. Asthma
4. Lowered blood sugar
5. Muscle loss
6. Dry skin
7. Weight gain
8. Lowered blood pressure
9. Darkened circles under eyes
10. Reduced sex drive

It is not necessary for you to exhibit all these symptoms to be diagnosed with adrenal fatigue. It is dependent on a lot of factors, such as the current stage of the disease, weight, age, and diet. It is recommended you write down whatever important or prevalent symptoms you experience so that when you visit the doctor, you will be better placed to explain yourself. This can also minimize your stress.

There are four general stages in adrenal fatigue syndrome. Each one has its own unique symptoms, which increase in severity from stage one to stage four.

The Four Stages:

1. **The Alarm Phase** – This is the first and most instantaneous response to a stress event. This stressful event can range from being admitted to the hospital, an exam, or an actual physical threat. When any of these things happen, your body begins to produce an extremely large amount of different hormones and neurotransmitters, such as insulin, cortisol, DHEA, norepinephrine, and adrenaline. All these chemicals are responsible for ensuring that your body handles the stressor in the appropriate manner. The majority of people who are in this first stage of adrenal fatigue tend to experience elevated levels of alertness and awareness, which then interferes with their sleep patterns.

The majority of people in this stage never notices or reports any symptoms, which means they probably spend their entire lives falling into and out of the alarm stage. Clinically speaking, there are generally no physiological or physical dysfunctions that can be pointed out during the alarm stage.

2. **The Continued Alarm Stage** – This is simply a persistence of the previous stage. The stress event continues as the body also persists in responding to the stressor. In this second stage, your endocrine system still produces the necessary hormones, but sex hormones like DHEA tend to drop rapidly. The reason for this is that the body is rerouting its resources toward production of stress hormones such as cortisol rather than sex hormones.

Another effect of the second stage is overworking of your adrenals. This is where you feel as if you are alert but tired at the same time. When this happens, some people start to rely on caffeine. During the day, the body may be alert but in the evenings you experience a sharp decline in energy. You begin to observe that you sleep more to recover from your daily fatigue. For women, menstrual irregularities and PMS can be experienced at this stage. Other symptoms that indicate hypothyroidism, such as slow metabolic rate and feeling cold also tend to show up.

3. **The Resistance Stage** – This third stage usually involves the continued production of stress hormones, which causes even fewer sex hormones like DHEA and

testosterone to be produced. The hormone that determines the development and progression of the resistance stage is known as pregnenolone. It is the hormone that is involved in the production of both stress and sex hormones, and its diversion is normally referred to as the "pregnenolone steal." People in this stage tend to be able to work and live normally, but the quality of their life is significantly reduced. Some of the symptoms that characterize the resistance stage include a reduction in sex drive, regular fatigue, infections, and feeling unenthusiastic. The body tends to accumulate toxic metabolites that cause insomnia and brain fog. The resistance stage may continue for months or sometimes years.

4. **The Burnout Stage** – As the syndrome persists, the body begins to get tired of the consistent production of stress hormones, thus causing the levels of cortisol to drop. With the reduction of stress as well as sex hormones, the body starts to give up and the sufferer experiences burnout. Some of the symptoms of this final stage of adrenal fatigue syndrome include apathy, irritability, no sex drive, loss of weight, depression, lack of interest in everything, and anxiety. Keeping a job and living normally becomes next to impossible for sufferers. This stage tends to be extremely powerful and devastating that overcoming it usually necessitates a total change in the sufferer's lifestyle.

The majority of sufferers tend to recover within the initial two stages of adrenal fatigue. This is the reason why you must find out the stage that you have reached in order to better determine the mode of treatment to be used to prevent the disease from progressing. The third stage is usually regarded as terminal because it involves your body switching of all its systems to divert energy toward survival. In stage three, your body cannot function properly all day regardless of how hard you try. Even a tiny stressor can result in a crash of your adrenal system.

The fourth and final stage normally constitutes an adrenal crisis characterized by pain in the lower back, vomiting, dehydration, and diarrhea. While some rush to the doctor prior to the onset of this adrenal crisis, others tend to ignore their condition until new symptoms arise. By this time, treating the condition becomes very hard and full recovery takes longer.

No matter which stage of this condition you find yourself in, there is always some form of treatment that can be used. Recovering from adrenal fatigue syndrome may be a long and arduous journey, but regaining your health and life is still possible. What you need to remember is that there isn't any single right way to deal with this condition. As long as you get to understand the stage of the condition you are currently in, you will stand a better chance of a complete recovery.

CHAPTER 2: FACTORS CAUSING ADRENAL FATIGUE

Though adrenal fatigue is today regarded as a silent epidemic, it is not a new phenomenon. It has actually been in existence since the dawn of humanity. The reason why it has become such a huge problem over the last century is because of the massive change in our lifestyles.

In today's society, stress levels and toxicity of the environment are extremely high. The diet we currently consume cannot be compared to what we were eating at the beginning of the 20th Century. Technology has played a major role in raising our stress levels, despite the fact that it is designed to make our lives easier and more comfortable.

It is very difficult to even get away and enjoy some peace and quiet thanks to our mobile devices. We are always engaging with our phones in one way or the other instead of just being present in the moment. The way we process and produce our food has been streamlined to the extent that more chemicals are being added to pre-packed meals. These chemicals were never present in our diet as we were evolving. Yes, technology and scientific advancements are great, but they also have many disadvantages.

The most fundamental reason behind every adrenal fatigue syndrome case is stress. In other words, the adrenal glands fail to deal with stress. There are some specific factors that must be considered in order to determine the cause of this condition, for example, the timeline. This condition doesn't just spring up overnight. It normally progresses over the years until it reaches the final two stages.

What this means is that in order to find out the type of stressor that started this condition, you will have to think about all the past stressors you have experienced. It can be simply one stressor or a blend of stressors. The truth, however, is that trying to remember the exact stressors that triggered the adrenal fatigue spiral is extremely difficult.

On the other hand, it would be of greater value to look forward to the future instead of focusing on the triggers of your stress. It is never a good idea to dwell too long on things that have passed. You will be better off pondering on ways of coping with future stress in a better way. Learning from past mistakes is one thing, but constantly worrying about them will only result in more stress.

Causal Factors:

1. **Emotional Stress** – Stress is widely regarded as adrenal fatigue's biggest cause. In most cases, stress creeps up because people assume they are capable of handling small stressors that affect them, not knowing that they actually have a long-term negative effect on the health. These stressors can include things like taking care of a new baby, sitting for an exam, or an unhealthy romantic relationship. These emotional stressors are all able to cause adrenal fatigue if they go unchecked for too long.

People face emotional stressors on a daily basis and they simply must learn to cope with them. Though there are times when people assume they're doing fine handling the stress, their bodies may be responding in an entirely different way, thus triggering adrenal fatigue. The problem starts when people stay in a stressful situation for an extended period of time, for example, sticking with an abusive relationship or working a stressful job. The body stays in a state of continual response to the stress, and before long, what appeared to be simply small stressors suddenly become too much to bear.

2. **Diet** – In general, your current dietary choices are much worse than they have ever been. You and most

people likely consume tons of pre-packaged and processed foods, and have abandoned vegetables and fresh produce. This is all down to the advancements in the technological capabilities that have given people the power to prepare food more conveniently. Nowadays, the average American eats 150 lbs. of sugar every year, yet only two centuries ago, it was a mere 1 or 2 lbs. Since your genetic structure didn't change over that short period of time, your body had to find a way to adapt to this drastic rise in empty calories. One of the ways of coping with the added sugar is to produce more insulin and cortisol, thus adding more pressure on the adrenals as well as the pancreas.

Another factor that can place added stress on your adrenals is obesity. Overweight people tend to consume excess calories, but most people fail to see the link between this and adrenal fatigue. Consider this for a moment; if you are overweight and are constantly tired, then it is obvious that your adrenals are also getting tired as well. In addition, overweight people suffer from anxiety and depression, both of which can lead to greater stress.

3. **Insomnia** – There are times in your life when you feel as if you are spreading yourself too thin. Achieving that balance between work and life becomes a

constant struggle, and there is simply not enough time to accomplish all that you want to. If this is the way that you feel, then it is likely that you are not sleeping enough. Ancient people used to sleep about 9 hours every night, yet most people today barely get half of that. On average, an American will sleep for 6.1 hours every night, and adrenal fatigue sufferers tend to sleep fewer hours than this.

It is through sleep that your body heals and recovers from all the stress faced during the day. The body has the power to heal itself, but you have to give it time. By sleeping fewer hours than required, you are denying your body this healing and recovery time, thus preventing your adrenal glands from functioning properly. It is recommended that you sleep for about 7 to 8 hours daily.

4. **Chemicals and Pollutants** – These substances exert a toxic load on the body. Toxic load means the toxicity level that you face every day. Examples of chemicals and pollutants you interact with daily include pesticides in food, chlorine found in drinking water, pollutants floating in the air, and antibiotics in meat. There are 2,000 chemicals that are being introduced into the consumer chain every year, yet the majority of these have not undergone any kind of testing to ensure they are safe for human

consumption. These chemicals go into the food chain while others are used to manufacture products people use. The result is the accumulation of these toxic substances in the body, leading to a compromised immune system, Alzheimer's, or even heart disease.

The majority of such kinds of chemicals have been proven to have a direct effect on people's adrenal glands. Though the human body is resilient enough to repair itself and adjust to the short-term implications, it cannot do this forever. In the long run, the stresses you place on the functioning of your adrenals starts to escalate toward adrenal fatigue syndrome.

5. **Chronic Disease** – Some of the stressors that can have a long-term impact on the adrenals are chronic ailments such as asthma, diabetes, and arthritis. There are diseases that place a huge demand on the adrenal glands - more than they can bear. This is especially true if you have been suffering from the disease for a long time. The medication that is administered to treat that disease may also end up overworking your adrenals, resulting in a combination of interdependent factors that trigger and catalyze adrenal fatigue.

6. **Trauma** – Adrenal fatigue can be triggered by long-term issues and not just short-term factors alone. In fact, a moment of an extremely traumatic occurrence

can be enough to cause a lot of adrenal damage. People generally assume that one moment of extreme trauma won't negatively affect someone, but studies are showing that the damage goes way beyond the superficial scars. Such moments can lead to long-term hormonal imbalance as well as reduced adrenal performance. This can also result from major accidents or even undergoing major surgery. This is why it is recommended that you take a good look at your personal and medical history when considering the causes of your adrenal fatigue.

The six causes outlined below are simply categories of what people believe are the major potential causes of adrenal fatigue syndrome. However, it is not easy to fully grasp the extent to which you experience these causal factors. If you look at modern society, you will realize that a lot has changed over the last five decades. Back then, getting a good job with no college education was possible, but today this is highly unlikely. A college degree is mandatory if you want to stand a chance of getting ahead of the competition. Not only is acquiring higher education stressful, getting a job after that and having to repay thousands of dollars in college loans can be extremely overwhelming. You have already stated that you may appear to be able to handle the stress adequately, but the fact is that your body may be struggling internally. The ultimate result is an accumulation of stressors and development of adrenal fatigue.

The biggest challenge people face is the way all these stressors are able to hide in the mundane aspects of daily life. They can be in the air or even the food. People now work longer hours just to pay the mortgage, and today a family with only one income will struggle with paying the bills.

The high level of consumerism that we have embraced as a society is also adding pressure to our lives. We have to keep up with our neighbors and friends if we are to be accepted, so we are forced to but the latest fashion in clothes and products. We take our work home with us and find ourselves still sending emails late into the night. The American way of life we live today is not the same as the one that existed five decades ago.

Stress can be found everywhere you look, so there is no way of escaping it. This makes it even harder to figure out the thing that triggered your adrenal fatigue, to begin with. A busier lifestyle means less sleep, and this cycle keeps going on and on. Smartphones and computers provide such a huge distraction in people's lives and just keep adding more stress on their bodies. It is clear to see that escaping stress in modern society is impossible.

Apart from the stressors you physically experience daily, there are also many virtual stressors as well. These are the "What ifs" of life, where you imagine hypothetical scenarios and how you would respond to them. The problem with imagined stressors is that the brain cannot differentiate them from real stressors, and simply responds to it in the same way it always does.

For example, if you are about to sit for a major exam, you will probably have to do a lot of studying, which can be very stressful. You are stressed about reading something and then forgetting it during the test, and your brain triggers a stress response. However, as you are about to fall asleep, you start worrying about the possibility of oversleeping and making it to the exam late. This virtual stressor causes your body to release more stress hormones, forcing it to also undergo additional stress.

CHAPTER 3: DIAGNOSING ADRENAL FATIGUE

It is not possible to make a diagnosis of adrenal fatigue syndrome using just one symptom or lab test. In order to enhance the accuracy of the diagnosis, medical experts must examine a variety of symptoms and perform numerous lab tests many times over. Patients are normally required to keep visiting their physician for a long time before their diagnosis is confirmed. Diagnosing adrenal fatigue syndrome is quite controversial because there are many doctors who refuse to agree that it is a real problem. This calls for extreme patience from the patient.

Some of the tests that are used to diagnose adrenal fatigue include standard hormone tests, which are conducted to confirm the level of thyroid hormones such as cortisol. There are also some tests conducted by integrative doctors and naturopaths. These kinds of tests are more focused on searching for neurotransmitters and hormones that will present a more accurate picture of the feelings the patient is going through.

There is great importance attached to your feedback to the doctor. You cannot rely solely on the tests because they sometimes give results that are within the normal range. It is only through regular interaction and feedback with your doctor that you can help them make an accurate diagnosis. This also helps determine the stage in which the adrenal fatigue may have progressed to.

Lab Tests for Adrenal Fatigue Diagnosis

1. **Cortisol Tests** – Checking the levels of cortisol in the body is the main test used to diagnose this ailment. It usually involves sampling the patient's saliva, urine, and blood. It is widely believed that sampling saliva is the best way to get an accurate estimate of levels of cortisol because that is where cortisol reactions happen. The patient is advised to drink water prior to the test since dehydration can interfere with the results. One sample is never enough. The doctor has to test samples all through the day in order to have enough results to compare. The reason for monitoring cortisol throughout a 24-hour period is because this hormone tends to peak in the morning and drop towards the evening. The doctor will try to determine the rate of decline as well as the presence of any spikes as the day progresses.

Interpreting the results of a cortisol test is not easy, and for this reason, it is recommended that you always consult a doctor who has prior experience with treating adrenal fatigue syndrome. Most labs tend to have a very wide range of test results, which means that doctors will only pay attention to those results that are considered abnormally low. This is why medical personnel avoids using the reference range and adopt optimal range instead.

2. **ACTH Challenge** – The aim of this test is also to confirm the level of cortisol in the body. In this test, the doctor will conduct a baseline test for cortisol and then inject you with the corticotrophic hormone. The aim of this injection is to get your adrenal glands to respond as they would during a stressful event so that the doctor can evaluate your stress response. If your adrenal glands release twice the normal amount of cortisol compared to the baseline test, then they are functioning well. However, if your cortisol levels don't come anywhere close to doubling the baseline level, then your adrenals may be impaired.

3. **Thyroid Test** – The human body is such a complex and interdependent system. In other words, your endocrine system is unable to function on its own without the other organs. Since the different systems in the body are connected to one another, a failure in one system will negatively affect the others. Research suggests that when the pituitary gland and hypothalamus become weak, then this could be an indicator of poor thyroid functioning. What this means

is that blood tests that indicate mild hypothyroidism simply mean that adrenal fatigue is responsible. There are a number of thyroid tests that are performed to determine the state of your thyroid. These include:

• **TSH (Thyroid Stimulating Hormone)** – As part of normal body functioning, your hypothalamus sends signals to your pituitary gland instructing it to produce TSH. This hormone TSH then instructs your thyroid to release T3 and T4 hormones. It should be noted that thyroid activity and TSH are inversely proportional. In cases where a patient's T3 and T4 levels are elevated, which is referred to as hyperthyroidism, then the level of TSH will be low. However, if a person is suffering from hypothyroidism (low T3 and T4), their TSH levels will tend to be high because their brain will constantly be instructing the thyroid gland to release hormones. This feedback loop is similar to what happens with cortisol and many other body systems. Adrenal fatigue sufferers usually have TSH readings that are way above 2.0 since their thyroid gland is not functioning, as it should. The TSH reference range is generally considered to be 0.5 to 4.5, and by looking at the reading of 2.0, it is clear to assume that the patient is within the range. However, they could still be suffering from an underlying problem, so the doctor must always consider this.

• **Free T3 and T4** – People who are diagnosed with hyperthyroidism are usually tested to determine their free T3 levels. On the other hand, this particular test is also helpful when trying to collect more information about the general functioning of your thyroid gland. Performing a free T4 test isn't common since the T4 hormone doesn't have as much of an impact as T3. Low production of T4 usually corresponds to high levels of TSH. These tests are designed to check for T3 and T4 that are 'unbound' and ready to be used immediately.

• **Total Thyroxine** – It is advised that this test be conducted together with the free T4 test. This is what will enable your doctor to determine the levels of T4 ready for immediate use and levels that are still bound to their carrier proteins.

4. **Cortisol/DHEA Ratio** – In this test, the doctor is able to determine how far your adrenal fatigue has progressed. In the first stage, both your cortisol and DHEA will be elevated. However, as the body continues to struggle to manufacture adequate stress hormones, the levels of DHEA will fall. This test is designed to check for the occurrence of the "pregnenolone steal." As the adrenal fatigue progresses into the latter stages, even the cortisol

levels will start to fall since the body is no longer capable of producing more of the hormone.

5. **17-HP/ Cortisol Ratio** – Cortisol is a byproduct of a material known as 17-hyroxyprogestrone. People suffering from adrenal fatigue usually exhibit greater levels of 17-hyroxyprogesterone compared to actual cortisol because their bodies are struggling to convert the raw material into the finished product.

The above tests are not the only ones that doctors can use to diagnose adrenal fatigue in patients. There are others that can be combined with the above tests, though they do not involve laboratory work. They are much less reliable than blood, urine, or saliva tests. Examples include:

6. **Postural Low Blood Pressure** – The normal reaction to a healthy person standing up on their feet is a rise in their blood pressure. Adrenal fatigue sufferers, on the other hand, will experience no change or even a drop in blood pressure. The degree of reduction in blood pressure indicates the severity of their condition.

7. **Iris Contraction** – In this test, doctors repeatedly expose the patient's iris to dark light in order to gauge the contraction. It is believed that a person with weak

adrenal function will not be able to keep their iris contracted for long.

There are some doctors who refuse to diagnose adrenal fatigue despite the prevalence of this condition. This is because they believe that these lab tests do not produce conclusive results. Labs tend to have reference ranges that are diverse from each other. The reference range is normally established by examining a segment of the population, checking the mean levels of their cortisol, and then setting the reference range 2 standard deviations from the average value.

Since cortisol levels often fluctuate as the day progresses, conducting tests at regular intervals within 24 hours can be quite effective. According to Labcorp, the cortisol ranges below are considered acceptable:

Morning hours: 0.025 mcg/dL – 0.60 mcg/dL
Noon: 0.01 mcg/dL – 0.33 mcg/dL
Afternoon hours: 0.01 mcg/dL – 0.20 mcg/dL
Evening hours: 0.01 mcg/dL - 0.09 mcg/dL

From the figures presented above, it is clear to see that the ranges are indeed extremely varied. If a patient has a cortisol measurement of 0.01 at noon, then they would be considered normal, but a cortisol of 0.33, which happens to be 33 times greater, would also be considered normal. If your level of cortisol at noon were to drop from the upper to the lower limit, it would be considered to be within normal range, yet this would represent a 97% drop!

For this reason, doctors and naturopaths use the optimal range instead of lab results. It should also be noted that the ranges for males and females are different. As long as the ranges are wide, doctors will have a tough time effectively diagnosing and treating patients. Doctors are not allowed to overprescribe medication to their patients, so how will they justify giving drugs to someone whose cortisol levels are considered to be within normal range? It is very important that you ask your doctor what their stand is within the first two weeks of visiting them. This will save you a lot of money and time.

In order to know which stage of adrenal fatigue you are in, doctors tend to use checklists. They note down your symptoms so that they can refer to them in the later weeks to determine whether you are stable or getting worse. The doctor must be a good listener if they are to detect your condition early enough. If adrenal fatigue is diagnosed late, recovering from it becomes that much more difficult.

There are also insurance and commercial challenges to the diagnosis of adrenal fatigue. The World Health Organization usually assigns a special code to each disease. This unique code is what insurance companies use to identify every disease that they cover. However, adrenal fatigue doesn't have a WHO code. Though doctors are still able to use the code that refers to "unspecified adrenocortical insufficiency," this move would be extremely challenging to support considering that the lab tests would bring results that are within normal range.

It may seem like a bureaucratic problem but if a disease doesn't have a code, then a doctor cannot send a bill to the insurance company. In other words, the doctor who diagnoses and treats you for adrenal fatigue doesn't stand a chance of getting paid. Another disincentive for diagnosing adrenal fatigue is the difficulty of its treatment. Effective treatment may require herbal supplements, changes to your diet, and sometimes hormone replacement. Most doctors find it more profitable to just treat your symptoms rather than have to deal with the underlying issues.

You must be willing to accept to pay for your own treatment, which can be extremely expensive. If you have enough money to pay for treatment without relying on an insurance company, then it will be much easier finding a doctor to diagnose and treat the disease. You can also choose to visit a naturopath instead, but you will still have to pay from your own pocket. They will still ask the same questions as a doctor, so be prepared to give honest answers. Ultimately, the best remedy for this condition is a natural recovery process.

The inability of the medical community to see diverse degrees is well known. A good example would be Addison's disease, which is an extreme form of adrenal insufficiency that is accepted by the medical world. However, adrenal fatigue, which happens to be a form of mild adrenal deficiency, is not considered to be a valid diagnosis. Some years back, it was difficult to diagnose someone with hypothyroidism if their test results were within the normal ranges, yet today, results close to the lower range lead to a diagnosis of mild hypothyroidism. It took two whole decades for this change to happen, so there is hope that adrenal fatigue will also evolve the same way.

CHAPTER 4: HOW TO RECOVER FROM ADRENAL FATIGUE

Estimates show that adrenal fatigue affects almost 80% of the world population. Some suffer short-term while others experience it over the long-term. You can succumb to stress in your daily experiences, but there are steps you can take to recover from this condition. The general steps for treating adrenal fatigue include reduction of mental and physical stress, adopting a positive mindset, and eating foods that are healthy and remove toxins from the body.

You didn't get adrenal fatigue overnight; so don't expect to recover from it that quickly. However, recovery won't take as long as getting the condition did. The human body has a huge capacity to heal itself if it is given what it needs. You have to provide the right conditions for healing to begin and sustain it, and as your health improves, you will realize that all the hard work was worth it.

Patience is one thing that you will have to hold on to because no silver bullet exists for treating adrenal fatigue. There are times when you will feel as if nothing is working, but if you maintain a positive mindset and change your lifestyle, you will begin to experience positive results. You may have to stop eating some of your favorite foods and start working out. Your recovery will be dependent on your level of dedication, perseverance, and effort.

Rules for Recovery:

1. Sleep

One major symptom that defines adrenal fatigue is tiredness even after a long night's sleep. As the condition progresses, insomnia is experienced. Therefore, an effective way to combat adrenal fatigue syndrome is adequate sleep every night. You will have to establish some kind of routine that you can follow. For example, set up a specific time to go to bed and remove all kinds of electronic devices from your room. With the incredible number of channels to choose from today, it is very easy to find yourself surfing channels till late in the night.

It is very easy to have your sleep interrupted by a beeping phone or tablet. Texts and notifications are always distracting you from whatever you are doing, so it is important that you switch off all electronic devices if you are intent on sleeping well. In case you need your device to stay on, then don't charge it in your room. Make sure that only emergency calls can get through and put it in another room.

Studies have shown that staring at a screen thirty minutes before going to bed interferes with the production of the sleep hormone, Melatonin. This hormone is what sustains your Circadian rhythm, and if you are watching something on a digital screen, then chances are you won't sleep well. You should also avoid waking up at night just to check your devices. Once you are exposed to a bright screen, going back to sleep will be difficult.

Your bedroom environment should have a relaxing atmosphere devoid of any light that may prevent your brain from shutting down. If necessary, get some dark curtains to block out any external sources of light. You could also invest in a good sleeping mask.

You also need to ensure that your bedding and mattress are comfortable and firm so you don't toss and turn throughout the night. If you can't afford a new mattress, then buy a memory foam pad to place over your mattress. Determine whether you are better off using pillows or not. Consider adjusting your bedroom temperature depending on your personal preference. Some people prefer a warm room while others want it a bit cooler. In case you have a sleeping partner, let them know what you plan on doing and ask them to accommodate your new preferences.

Avoid all kinds of noise in the bedroom. You can decide to close the windows, invest in earplugs, or if you can afford it, buy a white noise machine to block out unavoidable noises such as snoring. This machine can produce sounds mimicking a waterfall, rain, or even a fan.

It would be a good idea to develop bedtime habits such as checking the doors and windows, cleaning your teeth, saying goodnight to someone, and then getting into bed. Exercise can also help you sleep because expending energy tires you out and forces your body to demand rest. Try to find a simple combination of bedtime routines and exercise that can work for you.

2. Diet

The major defense mechanism that can effectively prevent adrenal fatigue is your diet. As you decide on how to use foods to support your recovery, there are two things you must consider: a diet that will help you recover and a diet that will make your condition worse. Meals should be consumed at the appropriate time and ensure you mainly eat whole foods. This may involve consuming a lot of vegetables and fruits and staying away from inflammatory foods.

Stay away from any food items you are allergic to since food sensitivities interfere with the body's ability to absorb vital nutrients. This may cause inflammation that quickly leads to interruption of your sleep cycle. You will then find yourself feeling weak and lacking energy. Just cut out all foods that you are even slightly allergic to.

Adrenal fatigue sufferers need to recognize that no other meal is as important as breakfast. Sleeping is the same as fasting for 8-12 hours, so when you wake up you need to refuel with the right kinds of foods. This should include mostly protein and a few high-quality carbs. For example, you could poach two eggs and eat them with blueberries, or eat a simple vegetable omelet. Do not continue partaking in the average American breakfast filled with sugary foods like waffle and cereals. If it comes in a box or packet, avoid it like the plague.

It will definitely save you a lot of time and money if you were to start preparing your meals in advance. You can make meals for the entire week so you don't have to make last-minute diet decisions. Go ahead and try out new recipes just to keep your diet interesting. Moderation is an important aspect of a diet; so don't eat too many sweet fruits since they still contain sugar.

It is recommended that people suffering from adrenal fatigue ensure they eat several small meals at regular intervals in order to maintain the levels of their blood sugar. Unstable blood sugar impacts your cortisol levels, so regular meals help prevent sugar crashes and cravings.

Consumption of excess sugar is known to place too much stress on the adrenal glands. Your energy levels may spike but this is soon followed by a crash, thus forcing you to resort to drinking caffeine to fight off the fatigue. Care needs to be taken these days because sugar is in all kinds of foods, even the healthy ones. Apart from the usual culprits such as cookies and cakes, fruit juices can also be a source of too much sugar. You are better off going for choices like beans, vegetables, and sprouted grains.

Proteins are a great source of energy that will last you much longer than sugary foods. For example, fish, free-range chicken, eggs, and beef are a great way to maintain high levels of energy for a long time. Always choose organic foods, not just because they are cheaper if bought at a local farmer's market, but also to avoid hormones and additives. When it comes to consumption of fats, always opt for healthy and whole options like seeds, cheese, butter, coconut, and dairy.

Water is a vital aspect of any diet, so drink water all through the day. Apart from what are considered traditional Western foods, there are some alternative foods that can aid in a speedy recovery. A good example is bone broth, which is known to be nutritious, lowers inflammation, boosts your immunity, and promotes healthy cholesterol. There are also fermented drinks such as kombucha and kvass that offer a variety of minerals for aiding digestion and absorption of nutrients.

Seaweed is a great option when it comes to intake of phytonutrients and minerals that can't be easily found in the traditional diet. Most supermarkets stock different kinds of seaweed so go for variety to maximize its benefits. You should consider shopping in different places especially traditional grocery shops and local produce markets.

Always keep an eye out for food labels, especially if you are buying something in a can. Avoid making assumptions that a certain type of food is healthy. There are a lot of hidden sugars and additives in prepackaged food. Just to be safe, always go for frozen or fresh produce rather than the canned variety.

Effects of Caffeine

Caffeine is an addictive stimulant that most people consume without understanding its full effects. It may begin as a benign attempt to get more energy but this is usually temporary. This leads to a continuous spiral of energy highs and lows, with every low stimulating a desire to drink more caffeine. Most people suffering from adrenal fatigue confess that as time goes by, the coffee they drink doesn't provide as much energy as it used to. This forces them to start drinking larger cups and consuming more sugary foods.

Every time you drink coffee, the brain tells your pituitary gland to release a hormone that triggers the production of adrenaline and cortisol. This leads to a stress response similar to that triggered by actual danger. The effects would be manageable if you are an occasional coffee drinker. However, if you tend to drink coffee all through the day, then your body will progressively weaken as your coffee tolerance increases. What is happening is that your body is now unable to handle the caffeine and you are weakening your adrenal glands.

What you need to do is immediately stop drinking coffee. Don't worry about the withdrawal symptoms that people talk about. These won't last more than a week. Sufferers of adrenal fatigue tend to experience greater energy levels after quitting coffee.

Coffee can be very addictive, and one way of giving it up easily is by opting for a decaffeinated version. The mode of preparation and taste is the same as before, except you will be spared the negative health effects. Since most people consider coffee their only way to wake up, you should try to wake your body up naturally by setting your alarm to go off 30 minutes early. Then drink some lukewarm water topped off with a lemon slice. This will stimulate and refresh you.

Instead of undergoing the headaches that are associated with caffeine withdrawal, you could try to reduce your coffee intake gradually. When the time comes to abandon it completely, stay strong and use your willpower to just say "No." Develop new routines that aren't related to caffeine.

Foods for Promoting Recovery

Now, let's focus on the foods that can help you heal faster. Vitamins are important, as are minerals. Consume foods containing B vitamins, more so pantothenic acid. Without adequate pantothenic acid, your adrenals shrink and weaken. B vitamins are also known to boost your energy levels whenever you are in a stressful situation. Examples of foods rich in vitamin b are bananas, potatoes, beef, legumes, oats, Brazil nuts, and turkey.

Vitamin C also plays a major role in helping the adrenals produce cortisol. During a stressful situation, the levels of vitamin C stored in the body's adrenals tend to drop faster than normal. This means you should make sure that part of your daily ration of vegetables and fruits include foods containing large quantities of C vitamins. These include asparagus, peaches, mangoes, tomatoes, broccoli, Brussels sprouts, citrus fruits, and spring greens.

Another vitamin that helps lower the stress placed on the adrenals is L-tyrosine. It helps in the transmission of signals from one body system to the next. Stress causes the levels of L-tyrosine to drop, thus making it paramount that you consume foods that replenish this vitamin. These include pork, oats, legumes, bananas, nuts, chicken, avocados, fish, whole grains, and seeds.

These are the foods that you need to keep on consuming to ensure that you have all the vital vitamins to fight adrenal fatigue. You can add some more to the list but the ones listed above are the ones you should focus on. You can eat them whole or make smoothies out of them.

Supplements

It is a well-known fact that adrenal fatigue leads to hormonal deficiencies. However, your body may also suffer from a shortage of other compounds, nutrients, and vitamins necessary for efficient operation of the body. While you may have discovered that your blood tests are within the normal reference range, this information is considered to be inconclusive. Just as it is important to maintain the optimum levels of your hormones, it is also crucial that your nutrients and vitamins are at optimal levels.

You can recover at a much faster rate if you take probiotics and herbs to help your body take in nutrients. It is important that you pay attention to what your body is telling you so that you can identify the right mix of supplements. Don't just take the same supplements that another person is taking. Recovering from adrenal fatigue is not about using the same treatment on different patients since it may work for one patient but not another. Ensure that the supplements you buy are of high quality and organic.

Most people suffering from adrenal fatigue tend to be deficient in vitamins, B12, B6 and B5. These need to be replenished through supplements. These vitamins are crucial in boosting metabolic pathways designed to elevate energy levels and minimize tiredness. Vitamin

B4 is responsible for helping in the manufacture of coenzyme A, an enzyme that is critical in the process of cellular respiration and breakdown of carbs, proteins, and fats. Vitamin B6 helps in the creation of adrenal hormones. Cell repair, red blood cell maintenance, and energy production are all supported by vitamin B12. These three vitamins are commonly combined into a single pill for convenience.

It is usually recommended that you take supplements for vitamin C because the vast majority of people fail to get adequate amounts of this powerful antioxidant from the diet. This vitamin is directly linked to the production of cortisol. It is required for adrenal gland recovery, and patients are usually advised to start with 1000 mg and then up the dosage gradually. Vitamin C should be taken with bioflavonoids.

Research suggests that an estimated 75% of people living in the United States are suffering from a deficiency in magnesium. This mineral is responsible for the regulation of energy flow around the body. This is an important aspect of trying to recover your health and boost energy levels. There are a number of symptoms that indicate a magnesium deficiency, including, depression, the stiffness of the muscles, cramping, and insomnia. On the other hand, be careful that you don't take too many magnesium pills otherwise you will experience digestive issues. It is recommended that you start with a 400 mg dose.

There are tons of scientific researches that support the use of probiotics as a way of boosting your health. They have been proven to lower stress, aid digestion, and minimize the negative side effects caused by antibiotics. By improving digestion, what you are doing is enlarging your body's capacity to absorb nutrients from your diet. The body is then able to heal faster, become stronger, and produce vital hormones. Your immune system is also strengthened through consuming probiotics. It is advised that you choose those probiotics that contain a minimum of 10 billion units and at least five diverse bacterial strains.

Most traditional cultures used herbs as medicine for hundreds of years. This is because herbs are able to help the body recover from adrenal fatigue. You can take herbs and supplements together if you want to boost your recovery. However, be advised that you do not have to take all the herbs that are listed below. Just choose those that you feel will work for you.

• Licorice Root - As an herbal supplement, licorice root is able to increase your endurance, trigger production of hormones, and keep your energy levels stable. People suffering from adrenal fatigue will love this herb because it aids in the circulation of cortisol in the body for extended durations. However, be warned that it also raises blood pressure, so if you suffer from both these conditions, stay away from licorice root.

• Ashwagandha – This herb performs diverse functions in the body, including lowering high cortisol levels, and raising low cortisol levels.

• Siberian ginseng – This herb is used by Russian Olympians to boost stamina, but it can also elevate energy levels and mental awareness. However, as with licorice root, people with high blood pressure should not use it.

• Maca root – Research has shown that Maca root is able to regulate cortisol as well as blood sugar. This herb also enables the hormones in the body to be absorbed by cells more effectively and efficiently.

• Omega 3 – The majority of people have adequate levels of Omega-6 in their bodies, but it is an Omega-3 deficiency that most people suffer from because the foods they consume don't have enough of it. This imbalance can easily cause inflammation that can only be managed by more cortisol production. Obviously, this creates added stress on your adrenal glands. In order to give your adrenals a lighter workload and minimize inflammation in the body, you should take Omega-3 supplements.

Make sure that you read every label of every bottle or packaging of supplements or herbs you take. Take the recommended dosage so that you do not suffer from any negative side effects. If the dosage is not well established, then use your body signals to determine how much works for you. Don't be in a rush to find the right herbs and supplements. Take the time to decide the best option for your condition.

Remember, as mentioned before, treating adrenal fatigue is more than just finding a single correct formula which works for everyone. Recovering from adrenal fatigue is a long-term process that requires utmost patience. Treatment can go on for months, so be prepared to take these supplements for a while if you want your recovery to be faster and easier. It must be noted that the supplements given here are not a cure-all in any way.

CHAPTER 5: ACCELERATING RECOVERY WITH LIFESTYLE CHANGES

Modern medicine tends to ignore the fact that your mind has power over your body. Recently, it has been proven that changes in your psychology can massively impact your physical health. One great example of how your mental state can stimulate diverse physical changes in your body is stress. Stress is able to affect every organ responsible for maintaining good health. If the stress is prolonged, then chronic adrenal fatigue can set in. That is why it is so important to tackle the underlying causes of chronic stress so that you can recover from adrenal fatigue.

Here are some of the ways to change your lifestyle in order to speed up your recovery:

1. Physical Exercise
When choosing the kind of exercise to perform, you should always consider the adrenal fatigue stage that you are presently in. The final two stages of this syndrome generally involve a lack of hormones necessary for engaging in strenuous activities such as soccer or running. This is because you will experience a severe drop in adrenaline once the activity ends. For this reason, you should choose low impact sports such as walking, yoga, or swimming. If you are still within

the initial two stages of adrenal fatigue syndrome, then you can do some weight training or run since exercise helps control your cortisol levels.

It is also advisable to engage in an exercise in the morning hours so that you do not risk disrupting your nightly sleep cycles. This will also boost your metabolism for the day. Older people cannot exercise for too long, unlike younger people, so just make sure that you don't exhaust yourself.

Avoid the habit of skipping your workouts because exercise is a great way to relieve stress. Make a schedule and stick to it.

2. Meditation and breathing exercises

Research has shown that through meditation, you can change your immune responses, brain waves, and circulatory patterns. Regardless of the stage that you are in, deep breathing techniques and meditation can help you. For people in the initial two stages of the syndrome, benefits include a reduction in stress levels and stabilization of cortisol and adrenaline. For those in the latter two stages, it will boost circulation and energy levels.

Sitting still for a whole two minutes may seem difficult, so expecting to meditate for 20 minutes can appear daunting. However, you have to focus on the many benefits you get, so take at least 15 minutes to sit down in a quiet place. It can be on a floor or chair, as long as you ensure a natural back posture. Shut your eyes gently and start taking deep breaths slowly. Inhale through the nose and exhale via your mouth. The initial breaths may be shallow but they will gradually get fuller and deeper. Pay attention to every breath as it enters and exits your lungs. If random thoughts come into your mind, just let them float by and keep focusing on breathing. This will definitely get easier with more practice. When the time is up, open your eyes and stand up slowly. Repeat this process one or two times daily.

3. Reducing Stress

There are a number of strategies that are effective for reducing your levels of stress. One of the best ways is to prepare for any stressors in advance. For example, in case you are attending a business meeting, ensure that your clothes are all laid out and prepare breakfast the night before. This will help you get enough time to gather your thoughts before the meeting.

You can also listen to some soothing music as you drive or ride to your workplace. You can even do some muscle relaxation techniques to relieve more stress. For example, if you are driving, you can hold the steering wheel as you flex your back, shoulders, and arm muscles until they start trembling. Hold for 45 seconds before releasing. The result will be relief all over your upper body, but be careful that you don't let go of the wheel.

According to Swedish researchers, floating in water can help the body relax and reduce the levels of stress hormones. If you cannot swim, then obviously you need to consider your limitations. Don't go in too deep or you will simply elevate your levels of stress.

Another stress coping mechanism is to focus on solving one problem at a time rather than allowing yourself to be overwhelmed by several problems. Discern between real and imagined problems because your brain responds the same way to both kinds of stressors.

If something is bothering you, write it down in a journal or on a computer. You can also talk to people close to you.

Try to stay as optimistic as possible by avoiding stressful language. Stress experts have determined that you will handle stress better if you focus on the things that work in your favor rather than speaking negative statements. Use the word "hope" rather than "expect."

Stress and anxiety tends to destroy your sense of humor, so laughing is one of the ways of keeping stress at bay. Go ahead and indulge in a good comedy or hang out with a funny friend who leaves you in a laughing fit.

Instead of spending your evenings venting to your spouse about all the negative things that happened, choose the positive things that happened and create a positive atmosphere. Adrenal fatigue is best overcome by maintaining a positive mind. This will help you keep an open mind necessary for making lifestyle adjustments. Negativity slows down your recovery, so just move on even after making mistakes.

The techniques described above can be used individually or combined to form an effective strategy for relieving stress. Meditation is usually advised for people suffering from adrenal fatigue, but each individual should practice it their own way. There is no silver bullet for recovering from adrenal fatigue syndrome. It may take a long time, sometimes between 6 – 18 months, and commitment to do the work. On the other hand, once you start to see some improvement, you will gain energy. Maintain this positive momentum toward your goals.

The rate at which you recover will depend on how severe your adrenal fatigue is and how willing you are to change your lifestyle. Severe adrenal fatigue generally takes longer to recover, but it is best to take your time and enjoy the process. Celebrate every small breakthrough rather than merely looking at the larger picture. Remember that your recovery journey can become quite difficult, but be patient and stay committed so that you can achieve smaller goals that accumulate into larger ones.

CONCLUSION

With the information from this book, you now have a path to recovering from adrenal fatigue syndrome. Now that you know what to do, go ahead and put in the work necessary to ensure that you get well.

Best of luck!

THANKS FOR READING

We really hope you enjoyed this book. If you found this material helpful feel free to share it with friends. You can also help others find it by leaving a review where you purchased the book. Your feedback will help us continue to write books you love.

The Smart Reads library is growing by the day! Make sure and check out the other wonderful books in our catalog. We would love to hear which books are your favorite.

Visit:
www.smartreads.co/freebooks
to receive Smart Reads books for FREE

Check us out on Instagram:
www.instagram.com/smart_readers
@smart_readers

Don't forget your 2 FREE audiobooks.
Use this link www.audibletrial.com/Travis to claim
your 2 FREE Books.

SMART READS ORIGINS

Smart Reads was born out of the desire to find the best information fast without having to wade through the sheer volume of fluff available online. Smart Reads combs through massive amounts of knowledge compiles the best into quick to read books on a variety of subjects.

We consider ourselves Smart Readers, not dummies. We know reading is smart. We're self taught. We like to learn a TON about a WIDE variety of topics. We have developed a love for books and we find intelligence attractive.

We found that each new topic we tried to learn about started with the challenge of finding the pieces of the puzzle that mattered most. It becomes a treasure hunt rather than an education.

Smart Reads wants to find the best of the best information for you. To condense it into a package that you can consume in an hour or less. So you can read more books about more topics in less time.

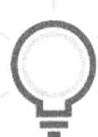

OUR MISSION

Smart Reads aims to accelerate the availability of useful information and will publish a high quality book on every major topic on amazon.

Smart Reads hopes to remove barriers to sharing by taking the copyright off everything we publish and donating it to the public domain. We hope other publishers and authors will follow our example.

Our goal is to donate $1,000,000 or more by 2020 to build over 2,000 schools by giving 5% of our net profit to Pencils of Promise.

We want to restore forests around the globe by planting a tree for every 10 physical books we sell and hope to plant over 100,000 trees by 2020.

Doesn't it feel good knowing that by educating yourself you are helping the world be a better place? We think so too…

Thanks for helping us help the world. You Smart Reader you…

Travis and the Smart Reads Team

WHY I STARTED SMART READS

Every time I wanted to learn about something new I'd have to buy 20 books on the topic and spend way too long sorting through them and reading them all until I arrived at the big picture. Until I had enough perspectives to know who was just guessing, who was uninformed and who had stumbled upon something remarkable.

I wished someone else could just go in and figure that out for me and tell me what matters. That's how smart reads was born. I want smart reads to be a company that does all that research up front. Sorts through all the content that is available on each topic and pulls out the most up to date complete understanding, then have people smarter than me package the best wisdom in an easy to understand way in the least amount of words possible.

For example, I got a new puppy so I wanted to learn about dog training. I bought 14 different books about dog training and by the time I got through the first 5 and finally started getting the big picture on the best way to train my puppy she had grown up into a dog.

Yeah she's well behaved. She doesn't poop in the house. I can get her to sit and come when I call. But what if someone else went in and read all those books for me, found the underlying themes and picked out the best information that would give me the big picture and get me right to the point. And I'd only have to read one book instead of 15.

That would be amazing. I would save time. And maybe my dog would be rolling over, cleaning up after my kids and doing the dishes by now. That my friend, is the reason I started smart reads. Because I wanted a company I can trust to deliver me the best information in an easy to understand way that I can digest in under an hour. Because dog training is one of many subjects I want to master.

The quicker I can learn a wide variety of topics the sooner that information can begin playing a role in shaping my future. And none of us knows how long that future will be. So why not do everything we can to make the best of it and consume a ton of knowledge. And I figured all the better if I can also make a positive difference in the world.

That's why we're also building schools, planting trees and challenging ideas about copyright's place in today's world. Because as a company we have to be doing everything we can to support the ecosystem that gives us all these beautiful places to read our books. Thanks for reading.

Travis

Customers Who Bought This Customers Who Bought This Book Also Bought

Natural Ways of Boosting Testosterone: How to Bulk Up and Put Your Sex Drive in Overdrive

Eating Clean: Detox, Reduce Weight, Fight Inflammation and Reset Your Body

Mint As Medicine: Discover The Powerful Healing Properties of Herb in Treating Headaches, Allergies, Asthma, Clarity and Peace of Mind

The Powerful Benefits of Myrrh: Effective Myrrh Recipes For Healthy & Beauty, Oil Pulling Therapy, Creativity, Aromatherapy and Improving The Mind

Probiotic Dieting: The Miracle of Probiotics in Healing Your Gut, Trimming Belly Fat and Weight Loss

Meditation Magic: Free Yourself from Worry, Depression, Stress and Anxiety

Meditation For Beginners: Overcome anxiety, relieve stress, fight depression, conquer fear, find inner-peace, happiness, mindfulness